Health
Made
Simple

BUILDING THE FOUNDATION OF HEALTH
THROUGH EASY AND SUSTAINABLE
CHANGES IN NUTRITION AND LIFESTYLE

BY JOHN SCHOTT

Schottswellness.com

Publishing services provided by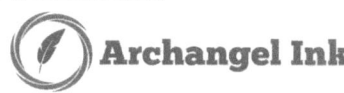

ISBN: 1517403812
ISBN-13: 978-1517403812

Table of Contents

4

Why This Book?

Being an active participant in the "health" field for nearly 10 years, I have studied, seen, experimented with, and learned a great deal from its broad canvas. Starting from a naive, extreme, and, yes, overly passionate advocate of the movement, to what I now consider a more mature and balanced-minded "motivator," I, too, have been exposed to the roller coaster ride that is the world of "healthy living."

The internet – via Google, social media, and an infinite number of blogs – has made it easy to access nutrition information and expand upon a growing food and health culture. Although it has created a positive influx of ideas, it has also created information overload that at times becomes quite contradictory and confusing. Should we eat low fat? Low carb? Vegetarian? Paleo? Are eggs good for us? What about gluten and dairy? Is there an agenda or commercial bias behind the answers to these questions? Is there a spiritual or moral dilemma involved? All these factors usually get us sidetracked away from tried and time-tested methods that revolve around our innate relationship with nature. We should consider slowing down and simplifying our lives in order to experience superior health and wellness.

Thus, the goal behind this book is quite easy. It is to harness 10 years of self-experimentation, and study and turn it into an uncomplicated and QUICK read. My hope is to "download" vast amounts of information and leave out all the superfluous details. The intent is to present a realistic and doable set of options that will enhance your overall whole-istic lifestyle. After all, we are beings with spiritual, emotional, electrical, chemical, and physical components that run as a fully integrated unit.

What you won't find here is the next big fad diet. You won't find someone endorsing anyone else's idea of the diet solution that will save the world and everyone in it. If I have learned anything, it is that there is no one program that fits into a nice little package that everyone can follow and succeed. I wish it were that easy. But many "authorities," health gurus, self-proclaimed experts and even scientists fail to see that there are so many complex layers involved in the whole equation. There are individual components that make us different. We need to consider lineage, epigenetics (our interaction with environmental factors), biochemistry & metabolism, and other lifestyle factors mentioned in this book. (Got sleep? If not, get some.) Besides, there are tools and great technological advances that can assist in individualizing your eating & lifestyle experience with proper testing (more on that later).

Our world is different than our Paleolithic ancestors. So is eating a so-called Paleo/ Primal diet appropriate? What about blood type? Although theories abound and seem promising, nutrition science is still in its infancy. These ideas have many questionable premises. All these different hypotheses, in my opinion, have come to us as a reaction to our involvement in an extreme, industrial, artificial, and experimental way of living our lives. So what's the solution?

Maybe it's time to go back to basics. Perhaps as we simplify and alter the way we live by blending time-tested ancestral practices with modern technological advances, we can attain a much-needed, balanced, responsible, and conscious wellness model.

So who am I to be dispensing this information? Why should my words even be considered to be a viable alternative choice? My primary drive has always been to assist and hopefully enrich the lives of all humans. I genuinely care for others. It may sound a bit esoteric or still a bit naive at times, but honestly, this is who I am. Again, after 10 years of being in the health field, I have taught nourishing cooking classes, done numerous consultations, given sound advice to thousands, and created a sustainable business model based on a successful whole foods organic restaurant that operated for five years. I have assisted many individuals in transforming their lives with safe and non-extreme cleansing programs and sound, time-tested eating strategies. And yes, I practice what I preach – albeit in a non-dogmatic, far-from-perfect manner.

And beyond all that, I also have an incredible opportunity. It is one where I can realistically help others see possibilities that emerge with a shift in perspective, and hopefully enhance their lives with just a few principles. For the last 40-50 years, we have been operating in an explosive and somewhat irresponsible manner. It has led to what can be considered a massive health crisis. One in three people (some experts say two) are estimated to face cancer today. Obesity, heart disease, diabetes, Alzheimer's, and so many other challenges are now being connected to lifestyle choices. People are following health advice from television commercials: ads created to sell billions of dollars in band-aid type drugs and products that mask symptoms and can have dangerous side effects. People are being told what to eat, not by their grandmothers, but by an industrial money-driven machine. This booklet can be a solid opportunity to improve your health. Take advantage of this valuable information created from many years of hardcore study and trial and success. ;)

I hope you can gain from this simple work as much as I have gained in all these years of self-exploration. If anything, just getting the Resources section, and using the links and recommendations there, will be enough to more than pay for this book. Dive in, enjoy, open your mind, and achieve your health sovereignty today.

John

Living Water: Human and Planetary Lifeblood

What is "living" water?

Living water is the vital lifeblood of the planet ... and of you. It is important to begin with this element in our discussion of primal wellness because—depending on age and other factors—we are designed to be 65-80% water. Living or "charged" water is crucial, as it directly interacts with our blood plasma, is seen in living ecosystems, and is the most natural.

Where can we find living water? The most ideal source of water is one that is wild and produced by nature--one created from deep underground aquifers untouched by pollution or human influence. It comes up through the earth in perfect form via true natural springs. There is an amazing free database that can point you to where these living springs have been located for collecting water. The site is findaspring.com. Not only does it offer vital information about current springs, but it is designed to be expanded with newly discovered access points to be shared and plugged into the site.

What's wrong with tap water?

Today's municipal water sources are lacking the intricate living elements and intelligence found in natural water. Most are improperly treated and infused with fluoride, chlorine, heavy metals, etc. They have a molecular structure that lacks a proper hexagonal pattern and its molecules are too large. All these factors make it difficult for the body to achieve proper hydration, transportation and assimilation of nutrients through cellular membranes, and miscibility with the blood. It also makes it more challenging to flush or wash out toxins from the body. Furthermore, most of these municipal water choices have a cationic or chaotic spin to them (down and out), which can create dysbiosis (improper bacterial balance), water retention, and overall biochemical disruption. All water is best consumed in an anionic pattern that's spinning up and in, with proper mineralization, and one that is totally free from toxins – thus "living."

What can we do if we don't have access to a spring?

In an ideal world, it would be best to drink water directly from a natural spring coming from an untouched deep aquifer directly as Mother Nature intended. Second best is perhaps a true well that is properly filtered with a coconut charcoal filter at the faucet. The key here is to do the best with what you have and upgrade as lifestyle changes and personal choices allow. So since not all of us have access to these choices, living in our technologically structured cities, it's important to be aware of and attempt to follow water's natural hydrological cycle, as much as possible. Charging water is a natural, energetic, and upgrading process performed on water in order to achieve the most absorbable, fluid, and useful water possible when access to a natural water source is not an option.

There are many ways of charging water, and some methods are more complex than others. The simplest way to make whatever water on hand somewhat charged is by starting with the purest water you can get, throwing a pinch of sun-dried sea salt in it (for a 16oz. bottle; or 1/3 tsp. for a full gallon, getting an ideal TDS reading between 85-140), and stirring it by hand with a wooden stick in a clockwise spiral. This water can then be enhanced by running it between magnets and leaving it overnight over lodestone and quartz crystals. Writing loving messages on the bottles doesn't hurt, either. ;)

Are there any purification systems you recommend?

After many years of water research, I have seen many great solutions to obtaining pristine, highly structured, oxygenated, sustainable, magnesium bicarbonate, living water from the convenience of your home. It is a technology called PristineHydro and it is convenient (check out the Resources section for the website).

The system being mentioned is beyond reverse osmosis (RO), distillation, water ionizers, plastic/stale/overly priced spring and other bottled waters. Once again, we are meant to be 65-80% saline solution water beings, so it is critical that we consider the best water strategy not only for drinking, but also for food preparation/cooking and bathing. Think about it in this way: if you take care of your water strategy, you're basically taking care of at least 65% of your overall health equation.

Should we drink the recommended 8 glasses of water a day?

The short answer is … it depends. Pay attention to your water needs. Too much water--hypernatremia--is quite real.

There is such a thing as drinking too much water, just as there is the more common chronic dehydration. Again, balance is key and no one formula fits all. Things to consider: height, weight, activity levels, how much other fluids you are taking, electrolyte balance. Are you eating enough salt? How much do you sweat? Are there enough minerals coming in? The Resources section has a few testing and individualizing techniques that can assist in finding the answers to some of these questions.

P.S. Stop drinking from plastic bottles right now. Get with the glass! :)

Remolding Emotions

This section is more of a long note rather than a whole chapter of sorts. It deserves mention from the beginning, as it's an area of great importance. It is an aspect of our lives that we tend to take for granted. As follows, I would like to invite you to surrender to past, present, and unforeseen future emotions. Simply understand that we are a species that is driven by e(energy in)-motion and there are elements of these unseen frequencies, vibrations, energies (or call them what you will) that get lodged into our tissues, electrical components, and overall mind-body connection. There is a ton of information that demonstrates how unresolved emotional issues from childhood, and beyond, play key roles in our physical and mental wellbeing. We have to be aware that these factors exist and can alter our health in many ways. So check out the Resources section for different avenues to release old emotional (stagnant) energy. There are great strategies and diversified methods that can assist anyone, based on what they are willing to do. If anything, at least become aware of the power of being present and that everything is a natural balance. Once we completely realize that we possess both all the "positive" and "negative" qualities in their entirety – and that we are both the hero and the villain – then we can achieve true freedom from emotions. We control them instead of them us.

Avoid the Die-t Trap

This section is the easiest to understand and quickest to grasp. It's also the one where most people find the greatest difficulty in changing. Again, too much complicated information overload out there.

But the bottom line is … STOP DIETING! Seriously, that's all that needs to be stated when talking about this particular subject. So honestly, skip the rest of this chapter now and get to the real density of the rest of this book.

However, if you're still reading this section, it's because – like me – you have a curious and strong desire to learn more. So I shall expand a bit upon my bold recommendation (bold especially in this society that is heavily conditioned to diet, diet, diet). There is big money in keeping people dependent on the yo-yo diet game and the endless sea of contradicting/confusing information attached to it. The diet war is definitely a causative factor of the disordered eating pertinent to us all living in the current century. This is why this chapter is necessary. I can easily leave you with the simple message delivered in the first few lines of this chapter, recommend a general foundation and ancestral approach of eating, and advise you to individualize your specific lifestyle and eating choices by using your own biofeedback mechanism as primary guide. I could even give mention to certain tests and technologies (more on this later) that can be useful, if necessary. Utilizing non-expensive yet efficient testing such as tissue hair analysis has an ability to pinpoint metabolic function, mineral balance pending on certain ratios, nutritional deficiencies, toxicity pertained to chemicals, metals, and/ or excessive accumulation of elements. It's quite valuable in streamlining someone's program and individualizing the experience. The truth, however, is that I want to emphasize how extremely skewed our view of dieting is. It really has become a disorder, and we must free ourselves of preconceived notions of one-size-fits-all, magic bullet, follow-the-guru approaches to eating.

Does a low-carb diet work? What about veganism, raw foodism, low-fat, Paleo, Pritikin, South Beach, or Jenny Craig? And the list goes on. The problem is that these diets all work for some people, some of the time. Here's the kicker, though – with all my years of health, nutrition, food, and dieting research, I've learned that THERE IS NO ONE DIET THAT WORKS FOR EVERYONE. There are elements that sometimes by chance align with your particular metabolism and offer some solution or advancement toward your health, but these are rare. This is where I believe we find the minority sect of diet gurus and evangelists who claim their dietary regime is indeed the one that everyone should follow, because they have found success with a particular way of eating. The problem is that their diet only works for them and a handful of other people.

I can say that from experience as I, too, was once such an evangelist. But, over time, wisdom and many kicks in the pants have balanced me out to be someone who can write this book with a balanced and strategic approach. After all, I'm not selling the next diet fad or urging you to subscribe to my billable program. As you'll see toward the end, you'll have a tool kit that can hopefully serve you to find the answer(s) that will best fit you and your particular lifestyle. Where we get into trouble with all the made up diets mentioned is when we begin to eliminate or drastically reduce a certain macronutrient, food group, or food prep mechanism (like cooking, in the raw food diets) long-term. We need all of it in its balanced way, at the appropriate time, and according to the way we live our lives today.

Like I mentioned in the introduction, we all have individual components and diverse metabolisms, ethnic backgrounds, mixed lineages, etc. So why are we so easily seduced by the next or previous "doctor" prescribed diet fad? I have a twofold theory: one, we are a symptom-driven, "want it now" type society that wishes fast results with very little commitment and effort; two, we are constantly bombarded by major media messages feeding us false perceptions of beauty, while ironically pushing addictive, excessive, calorie-laden fast food. This paradox keeps us in the vicious cycle of gaining weight while wishing that we looked like the photo-shopped supermodels. If that's not insanity, I don't know what is. Want to go further? The same clique of folks who benefit from the billions made by these two dietary and media avenues will gladly gang up on us by telling us that what ails us is quickly and easily solved by the next pharmaceutical drug that, oh by the way, has a laundry list of side effects that nobody really knows much about. See how deep the rabbit hole goes? I'm not doing this to scare anyone; I simply want to highlight that there is indeed a Diet trap out there. Don't fall for it! Instead, eat real food.

Nourishment: A Primal Foundation

What is nourishment?

nour·ish·ment
/☐ n☐ riSHm☐ nt/

Noun

> The substances necessary for growth, health, and good condition.
> Food.

Synonyms

nutrition - food - nutriment - aliment - sustenance

So, if we were to simply go by that definition, the whole eating paradigm should be quite simple. And it is. The bare bones answer is to eat that which we recognize as "real food." These are elements that ideally come from nature, which nowadays has been morphed into something else. So it leaves us with a more complex idea of what to use for nourishment, and thus the premise of this particular chapter.

Eat the Food: what's in and what's out?

We have evolved into our current brain size, species behavior, and physiological progression, primarily as a hunter-gatherer society. So, what do we hunt? Animal protein of different sorts (wild game, fish & seafood, beef, poultry, pork). And what do we gather? Fruits, vegetables, eggs, nuts, seeds, root vegetables, and tubers. You may be thinking at this point, "Oh no, all this preface, only to get to yet another primal/paleo diet? Here we go ..." But not really. The list mentioned above consists of a strong foundation – a program that presents a solid basis of nourishing, nutrient-dense, and calorie-appropriate foods. It's where most of the consistency is to be highlighted. Today, we can also take it a bit further and, for some, possibly include some high quality full-fat dairy, legumes, and, under the right circumstances, certain whole and ideally wild grasses (grains).

That being said, there has to be some mention of some "foods" that should be considered rare options and/or avoided altogether. These come mostly from laboratory settings where humans, not nature, have attempted to improve the food supply and, so far, fallen short of the mark. I'm talking about the major culprits behind many of our major health challenges today.

White Refined Foods

Here, I'm not talking about natural and legitimate white foods such as cauliflower, yucca, and grass-fed cultured live yoghurt. The main players here are white sugar, white flour, white factory-farmed, pasteurized, homogenized dairy, and, to some degree, white table salt. These all have been suspected to be related to increasing inflammatory pathways, raising insulin, and causing sugar spikes, as well as being some of the most common allergenic, immune-suppressing substances.

Again, this doesn't mean that all white foods are unacceptable. Here's where the nutrition world gets into extreme notions of what's "good" and what's "bad." There is context for all things. For instance, take the ample consumption of white rice in most Asian cultures and what seems to be no ill effects directly from it. This is contrary to the "brown rice is healthy" idea that, for many, has shown to create digestive issues spanning from knee and joint pains, all the way to irritable bowel. Does this have to do with the fact that white rice is missing the bran and fiber component and is thus easier to digest? Both seem to offer the same nutrient profile, which is generally low to none, so then why eat it in the first place? For some carbohydrate-dominant folks (as per biological/chemical typing) and athletic folks, white rice can be an easy-to-digest complex source of fuel that the body can handle well. Add to it mineral-rich broth (the real stuff, not the thing that comes in a tiny packet with "natural flavors") instead of just plain water, and you have a now improved, nourishing product. It's all in the details and in learning to adjust the culinary element accordingly.

Gluten

The term "gluten-free" has become synonymous with healthy, and is possibly the fastest-growing diet trend (fad?) on the market right now. For those of you who don't know, gluten is a complex protein found primarily in wheat, but also in other grains like barley, rye, spelt, kamut, and triticale. Gluten has been highly recognized as one of the most allergenic, immune-suppressing foods. Numerous people have also shown ill effects, digestive issues, and ongoing aches and pains due to the possible inflammatory action that this protein can create. Although it is indeed an issue that deserves to be looked into, not everyone (as some people will lead you to believe) is gluten intolerant or gluten sensitive. Proper testing for this is tricky and complex, but if your body is hinting that it is affecting you, it may be worth the investment. I typically stay away from it, for the simple fact that today's wheat products are significantly different than the wheat of old (known as Emmer or Einkorn) that we evolved with for most of our history. Today's wheat has been extremely hybridized and genetically modified, and the gluten component has been concentrated beyond its natural state. If you do wish to consume wheat, you can consider the proper handling of the grain, which usually consists of soaking, cooking, and fermenting. Alternative grains such as rice, quinoa, buckwheat, and millet do not have gluten and may be worth exploring. The least that can be done is to take your pulse before consuming wheat by itself, and then 15 and 30 minutes after, to see if it is significantly elevated. An elevated pulse would indicate that the body views the gluten-containing grain as a stressor. The other alternative is to go on an elimination diet and reintroduce one item at a time to see how your body reacts.

Dairy

The concept of drinking supermarket milk that comes from other animals is an idea we've long been sold by an overly marketed dairy industry – a "cash cow" if you will. On the other hand, we've been drinking real milk since we moved into an agricultural model some 10,000+ years ago. So here, we're going to put a few concepts on trial and hope to make the best educated decision possible when it comes to choosing this category of foods or not.

In order to not get too deep into the issue of whether we ought to drink milk or not, here are a few things to consider:

1. Cows drink milk from cows. Humans drink milk from humans. We are the predominant species of mammals that has developed a consistent practice of drinking milk from another species. But then again, we're the only species driving cars, wearing shoes, and cursing people out in heavy traffic. ;) So with that, all philosophical perspectives get skewed and thus lead to the conundrum.

2. Cows' or another animal's milk is meant to be taken by a baby of that same species in order for proper growth periods (spurts) to take place. Again, our species seems to be the persistent one attempting to carry on a practice of drinking milk beyond the allotted natural time period.

Noting these first two points, however, it's possible that you could fall into the category of those people who have become what we call lactose or dairy persistent. These are, believe it or not, folks who have actually developed an epigenetic capability to properly digest, assimilate, and utilize high-grade qualities of milk to their benefit – especially with things such as kefir, raw butter, and other cultured products such as yogurt, cheese, and buttermilk. Find out where you lie in this spectrum, make the appropriate choice, and you may be able to use some or all of these products to some advantage in your nutrition plan.

3. Casein is a major (theoretically indigestible) protein found in milk products that can be very difficult for the body to break down, and can create an ongoing inflammatory, mucus- and acid-forming situation for our body terrain. Now, is this solely applicable to pasteurized, homogenized, factory-farm dairy where these elements are the major culprit to the denaturing of such protein? Or does it apply to grass-fed raw dairy, as well? These are all things to explore and consider.

Also, there may be different forms of casein that may be digestible depending on the grade of milk and type of ruminant (cow vs. goat, for example, or even Holstein cows vs. Jersey cows). Once more, this is personal homework to experiment with, as different varieties may be fine for some people.

4. Raw vs. cooked milk: does it matter? When it comes to dairy products, the whole pasteurized vs. raw seems to be not only very controversial, but also quite significant. If someone does choose to have some dairy as part of their lifestyle, then raw from a free-range, grass-fed animal seems to be the most optimal choice (again, just be mindful of all the other reasons to consider before deciding whether this food is for you). Why raw? This form of milk is loaded with enzymes such as lactase, which predigests the lactose. This means that in cases of people who believe that they are lactose intolerant, the raw milk may be digested and true intolerance is not applicable. Another advantage to fresh raw milk is the probiotic element found in the food. This also assists with digestion and the development of proper gut health. Lastly, full-fat whole milk and its byproducts are the way to go, as it seems that the magic is in the fat.

A note on calcium: Not all calcium comes from milk (although it is a good source). So if this is not a workable choice for you, here's some comfort. There seems to be plenty of ASSIMILABLE or bioavailable calcium from leafy green vegetables that have enough alkaline minerals that – if consumed with enough fat and a well-rounded program – present enough calcium for many. Also note that a combination of collagen-rich amino acids and bone-building protein with magnesium in the form of bicarbonate (homemade bone broth!) may be the bone-building strategy you're looking for.

Sugar

Sugar has recently been made out to be the worst of all "devils." But don't go on a low-carb diet just yet. The data that the low-carb diet camp has focused on is mostly considering one hormone – insulin. Once again, the diet industry has gone to extremes. It turns out that we run on a spectrum of different hormones, not just one, and additionally, not all carbohydrates are the same. Typically, when we limit ourselves to whole food carbohydrates (bearing in mind our individual biochemical type) like fruits, vegetables, tubers, root vegetables, and a few whole grains here and there, we will typically be set on the "sugar" carbohydrate front. Where we may run into trouble is when we unnaturally concentrate a substance beyond its biological use – in this case, processed white sugar, high fructose corn syrup, and excessive amounts of fruit juice. Keep in mind – when consumed occasionally, these can temporarily raise metabolism and create an anti-stress effect. But generally, we are best served by incorporating some natural whole food carbohydrates within our individualized balanced program and avoiding the refined sugars. We have evolved eating these natural carbohydrates, and our brains run optimally on glucose.

What about artificial sweeteners?

Artificial sweeteners such as aspartame, sucralose, neotame, acesulfame potassium, and saccharin seem to be even worse than sugar, itself. I would avoid them.

Rancid Oils

I'm talking primarily about hydrogenated and partially hydrogenated vegetable oils here (PUFAs). These are substances like canola (rapeseed), corn, soy, and cottonseed that go through an elaborate process to achieve deodorizing, shelf life, and desired consistency. (Can you say plastic?) The short of it is that these are extremely oxidized, rancid oils that are very disproportionate in the amount of omega 6 fatty acids (too high) vs. omega 3s, which creates a highly inflammatory condition inside the body – not good news. My money's on these to be the major causative factors for the modern high incidence of heart disease and NOT saturated fat and cholesterol. It's best to go the traditional route by using cooking oils that are heat stable and nutrient rich, such as coconut oil, ghee or real butter, olive oil, palm oil, and tallow.

Other ingredients to be extremely mindful of are herbicides, pesticides, preservatives, fillers, and food coloring. All of these are chemical, laboratory-made substances designed to magnify taste (MSG), extend shelf life, and create convenience when manufacturing. These are alien to our biology and can create toxic loads in the body, and disrupt a great deal of the body's normal functions. Other examples of questionable food additives are the nitrates and nitrites found in processed meats, which also present a great deal of health challenges when consumed.

GMOs *(Genetically Modified Organisms)*

There is a great deal of controversy with this topic, as of this writing. The pro side sees it as a potential to create more yield and thus feed the whole world; the against camp claims that they are unsafe and can cause major health problems. The way I see it is that this is yet another way humans try to improve upon what's natural, which we don't have a great track record of success with. The jury is still (sort of) out on the safety of these foods, and there is lots of potential evidence that points in the direction of them being dangerous. For now, my recommendation is to avoid all GMOs until we have solid, non-biased, clinical trial-based evidence. This is probably unlikely to happen, so for now (and maybe forever), great caution is truly advised.

Soy

Soy – especially tofu, soy milk, isolated soy protein, and mock meat products from soy – is not only mostly GMO, but has also been shown to be a highly difficult-to-digest food. Soy products present endocrine disrupters, high levels of phytoestrogens, and isoflavones that create great hormone imbalances in both males and females. Eating soy can feminize men and increase cancer, and also create an overly masculine condition in women. In an attempt to "combat" heart disease and promote a "healthy" vegan diet, soy has been the champion for these causes, but soy has never been utilized as a food to the extent that we use it in the West. I would seriously reconsider this choice or at least do some further research. Traditionally, soy has been used mostly as a condiment and/or supplemental cultured (fermented) food such as natto, miso, real tempeh, and Nama shoyu. Check out the Resources section for more information and links on soy.

To summarize this section, eat real whole food and culinary offshoots of real foods that can be recognized by your human biology. Use the traditional eating approach as a foundation and, ideally, eat based on properly-tested biological metabolic typing (see Resources). Stay away from the main red flag foods mentioned above, and don't stress too much about diet fads/ideas. Eat wild as much as possible, learn herbs, shop local, and see what your specific environment has in store for you. Magic happens when we eat in accordance to our unique local environs!

Cleansing & Detox: A New Perspective

The idea of cleansing and detox has been a growing trend in the health field that has also gained mass appeal – from celebrities doing the Master Cleanse (not a good idea) to juice cleansing operations that seem to be doing well as a business model. The thing to understand about the concept is that if the body is functioning optimally by running on the proper fuel, managing sugar/insulin properly while attaining a balanced PH and supporting your metabolism, no specific detox protocols are typically necessary. By eating the right foods based on your specific biochemical type (feeling), using individualized and proper supplementation, and following the other lifestyle elements laid out in this book, your body is more than equipped for handling elements that don't belong there.

A nutritionally based, safe, non-extreme, non-depleting, and short-term fast or cleanse every once in a while can be a nice change of pace, however, and, at times, even an additional aid to healing faster. But this should only be done with proper consulting and by being mindful/specific of your individual needs, in order to keep the body optimized. There are other factors that once in a while need to be addressed when the general food and lifestyle approaches based on biochemical blood work fall short. These incorporate issues involving heavy metal toxicity (e.g. metal amalgams in the mouth), severe infections, and other toxic elements coming from concentrated sources. There are other protocols that can be used with the help of a properly-trained individual or holistically-minded practitioner that can serve to assist with detoxification when necessary.

There is one more aspect with this subject that needs mentioning because of the time and environmental alterations we have imposed upon the planet. It revolves around the reality that our environment is no longer a pristine, biodiverse, balanced ecosystem, as compared to that which our ancestors inhabited. We are faced with challenges of excessive pollution, acid rain that has changed the state of rivers, lakes, and all bodies of water, chemicals in the food, depleted soils, excessive medication and drug use, off-gassing VOCs, and other elements such as electromagnetic frequency "pollution." Other aspects also come into play, such as ongoing nuclear fallout, excessive use of plasticizers, and other factors that escape our awareness because we have yet to really grasp the consequences of our abusive relationship with nature. These are aspects of our current environmental reality that need a modern strategy for proper adaptation. Therefore, in today's day and age, I highly recommend the use of inactive (non-exercise-induced) sweating via far or near infrared sauna as a weekly and ongoing practice. Other safe elements that one can incorporate as well are the practice of daily dry skin brushing with essential oils, using a neti pot, flossing and proper dental hygiene, and even rebounding to promote proper lymph movement. Furthermore, the use of edible clays – in specific cases, zeolites – and as much antioxidant foods and superfoods (more later) as possible are all considerations toward the overall health/detoxification strategy.

To end this chapter, please do your research before embarking on the next juice fad diet, master cleanse, water fast, or anything that is **extreme** and touts over the top benefits without any true scientific backing. Empower your immune system with the right nutrition, supplementation, and lifestyle modifications, and allow your body to run efficiently – the way it was designed to. And if you absolutely must do a cleanse of sorts, then I recommend doing a blended nutritional "fast" that takes your individual biochemical metabolic needs into consideration. To learn more about this option, check out the Resources section at the end of the book.

Beyond Nutrition: The Rest of Your Life

This is one of my favorite sections because it's highly underrated, but of extreme importance in the whole health equation. These lifestyle factors are some that take very little effort, but produce a great deal of value. Following will be a section by section, and short and sweet introduction to each area. You can deepen these as far as you like and as much as lifestyle adaptation/habits allow.

Stress Management

Stress is possibly the most taxing and detrimental of all lifestyle factors that challenge our well-being. It encompasses anything from constant financial worry to difficult relationships, overtraining, working too much/not playing enough, not having enough "free" time, and simply creating pressure situations that never get shut off. Other stressful elements involve the unnatural way that we live our lives. So what's the solution? There are many. Whatever relaxation and stress-management technique that works for you and that you will realistically incorporate is the best one. For some people, that's yoga; for others, it's meditation, visualization, going for a hike, swimming, taking up a hobby where your brain is shut off, seeking spiritual endeavors, or even spending time with a group of close friends and family where nothing "serious" is discussed. All these are fair game, viable, and effective. No matter what you choose, the key is to make time and the habit of reducing the excessive cortisol, adrenaline, and constant grind state that we live in. This leads to the next theme: sleep – possibly the most powerful anti-stress mechanism we have.

Sleep

The key is to achieve an average of 7-8 hours of deep and good, rejuvenating sleep every night. Anything under 7 or over 9 hours will typically become counterproductive to steady-state energy throughout the day. There is an incredible amount of data and science on proper sleep. If you would like to further understand the relevance of a good night's sleep, check the Resources. For now, the goal is to create great sleeping habits. Sleep is the number one anti-inflammatory agent. This is why you want to be in a cool(ing) environment while you sleep. Setting a proper sleep atmosphere is key, and it involves total darkness, no electromagnetic pollution of any sort, and reducing or shutting off lights and computer screens two hours before you go down for the night. Additional technology that can be beneficial includes changing light bulbs to low blue light (ideally LED) bulbs, and/or using special glasses that eliminate the blue lights from TV and computer screens. These artificial lights from electronic devices typically fool your body into thinking it is still daylight, thus throwing off our natural circadian (solar) rhythms, which flip our natural hormone progression and interfere with sleep.

Exercise

This area, much like the diet world, is filled with controversy and conflicting information. Is Crossfit good? Bad? Practical? Are weights the way to extend lifespan and remain strong? Will body-weight exercises suffice? Will long-distance endurance training (a la marathon running) make you look like a stick figure that has no muscle and is so stressed that a common cold takes you out in a second? Yes, ladies and gentlemen, there is such a thing as over-training, and exercise can be both a curse and a blessing. This is the complex nature of all things "healthy."

So with that, let us put a few things into perspective. My general view on exercise is pretty simple – do something you love, that you are willing to do without forcing yourself, and that involves natural, safe (injury free) movements. Then, rest and recover appropriately and don't overdo it. Oh, and make sure that you are in a strong metabolic state before doing too much intense training. This includes simple things such as having proper 97.8- 98.2 degree body temperature first thing in the morning and throughout the day, having warm extremities instead of ongoing cold hands and feet, making sure your energy is a steady state, erratic mood swings are limited or non-existent, and have strong digestion where there is no excess gas, bloating, and inflammatory discomfort. All these tend to be easy to self-monitor, and indicative of someone who can take on proper training. Remember, exercise makes a strong person stronger and a challenged individual sicker.

Things to consider when taking on a program: What is your goal? Are you getting enough sleep? What are your levels of stress in other areas of your life? Are you strong (metabolically) and healthy enough to add negative (excessive) stress on the body? How much time is available?

These are all elements that must be considered. You may have to consider working "in" before you work out – this is more along the lines of yoga, tai chi, and slow movement types of exercises. Rebounding on a high quality rebounder or trampoline is one of the very best whole body/cellular exercises anyone can do. Rebounder too expensive? Get a pogo stick. :)

The following is what I do right now. So far, considering my lifestyle and time constraints, this approach has kept me fit, as close to ideal body shape and content. My lineup is 2.5 minutes of all-out bike sprints 3 times per week, with Isometric exercises 2-3 times per week. I throw in some push-up, bar/pull-up work, and hanging yoga swing work in between all that, as well. And I love to do MovNat type drills, too. It's more like play and makes me feel like a kid. Check Resources for these. Don't sit for too long, and don't stand for too long – balance your ongoing movement. Don't ever underestimate rest and recovery. Finally, don't take walking for granted. It's impressive how fit one can remain by keeping your daily steps high and fine-tuning your eating.

Bodywork

Most of us think of bodywork and immediately think massage. Although massage is indeed a great tool for stress management, relaxation, and moving lymph and other energies in the body, there is also the kind of bodywork that involves more depth, and is a safe and effective way to break down scar tissue and re-strengthen the body – think Maori healer (romiromi massage). The techniques involved – sometimes involving pounding and mashing – are meant to work on loosening the body so that it symbiotically works in conjunction with the nutrition program. Other similar modalities involve trigger point, resistance stretching, foam rolling, Thai yoga massage, Ki Hara, and more (see Resources). Lastly, look into Vibram 5 Finger shoes. This is a bodywork tool of a different type, but quite powerful. Our natural design is to be barefoot. By getting into a constrained situation day in and out with any body part – in this case, the foot – the muscles, joints (metatarsal/ phalanges), and general structure will tend to atrophy. When the foot is in a cast of sorts (such as wearing the conventional poorly-designed shoe) or even a peg leg type model (high heels), we are restricting its natural ability to function within its complex range of motion. In many ways, we also lose our connection to the Earth and rest of the body. We were designed to walk for significant distances. Having the right working "equipment" – a la bare feet or the Vibram barefoot hybrids – makes a big difference in keeping all body parts working optimally. So get bare footing, wear more five finger shoes, and get over the whole arch support fallacy ;)

Grounding/EMFs

The idea of grounding is to simply reconnect with the natural electromagnetic charge of the planet. This type is healthy and meant to dissolve excessive amounts of positively-charged electrons ("unhealthy") that we are bombarded with via cell towers, phones, microwaves, and other elements of the technologically driven society. Although there are some potentially valuable technologies that work to ground us or align us more with the healing frequency of the planet (check Resources), the most effective way to take advantage of the negative electron power – possibly the most effective source of antioxidants – is to simply take your shoes off and plant your feet on the earth. Whether it's on the beach, in the forest, or even in a park where there is sand, soil, or earth of any kind, this free stream of healing/recovery energy is not to be taken for granted. Also, don't put the cell phone next to your head or wear/carry it anywhere on your body. Invest in a headset (and that doesn't mean a Bluetooth – these are worse). Check out the Resources section for more information on the science behind grounding.

Creating a Safe Home Sanctuary

This section focuses on what's in our surroundings. Although we have little control over huge factories, endless waves of car exhaust, and nuclear fallout, we do have complete control over our interior environment: OUR HOME. Optimizing our home into a safe non-toxic habitat may require an alternate perspective that involves diverse ways of living. Here are some ideas:

Be mindful of chemicals coming from off-gassing paint, perfumes (plug-ins), harsh cleaners, and excessive use of bleach. Soaps, detergents, and other disinfectants should be as natural, mild, and safe as possible. Limit or bypass the carpets and heavy drapes. These have a strong tendency to not only hold dust mites, and off gassing particulate matter, but also will accumulate higher incidences of bacterial and mold toxicity. Shower filters are great to reduce the chlorine from the tap. Invest in an air purification (HEPA)/ionizing unit that will keep the internal breathing atmosphere in good working order. And while you're at it, get some plants, open a few windows, and get some MOSO bags (see Resources). Please transition away from plastic toys for your children and invest instead in toys made from wood and natural materials. The BPA and plastics absorb through the oil of the skin and can wreak havoc on the endocrine system – this is no joke, folks. The extensive Resource page for this section is quite valuable and quite fun.

Also remember the EMF pollution. Turn breakers off where you can, throw out your microwave (or at least unplug and not use), and turn the wireless off at night before you go to bed.

Superfoods for Super Health

"Superfood" is a term that's become quite popular. Depending on who's defining it, a superfood can be anything from Goji berries to wild salmon, wild blueberries, dark chocolate (cacao), coconut oil, spirulina, and bee pollen. Some even consider kale (a nice veggie to have, but a superfood?) to make the cut. But before we begin to get more carried away (and yes, even possibly step into the realm of faddism), let's define terms. Again, a little perspective goes a long way.

A superfood, simply stated, is a food that can offer high concentrations of nutrient density, borders the line of being medicine, and offers a high spectrum of different constituents, making it a potentially superior substance to everyday foods such as the humble tomato. So in some ways, a few of these foods are special. We must consider, however, that when it comes to calorie density and whole body nourishment, these so-called superfoods are still simply add-ons. To attempt to fulfill our dietary needs with this genre of food alone can both create excessive concentrations – leading to possible toxicity – and malnourishment. No matter how many claims about nutrient density and off-the-chart benefits a diet guru makes, these aren't the be-all and end-all. For instance, let's take cacao (chocolate). Although cacao is very high in magnesium, chromium, and antioxidants, and has constituents that make people feel good, it can also be highly stimulating. It can be addictive, a potential adrenal suppressant, and can keep you up if you're sensitive to theobromine and caffeine. It has its place, like all the other superfoods, and it is meant to be used wisely.

Because of their high value, if money and time allow you to incorporate some of these items into your lifestyle, do it. And although not many scientific double-blind studies have been done that can provide evidence that they will in fact do wonders for the body, there are several superfoods that I do believe are worth looking into. So with that, I will share my top choices and the ones that may deserve a little bit of investment. The following list has been chosen because it has a solid combination of time-tested traditional use blended with technological advances. Since this book is meant to be a quick read and one to lead you into further exploration, I will take my top choices and quickly share why they have been chosen. Here we go:

Marine Phytoplankton

Or more accurately, the suspended living seed of the ocean. This is where the most compatible strand to human DNA of a plant source, Nannochloropsis Gaditana, has been extracted properly via technological means. It's pure energy in a bottle that feeds your mitochondria and enhances neurotransmitter activity.

Seed Oils

The combination seed blend of this specific product (due to the technological advancement in the extraction of these oils/juices) from Sunflower, Flax, Black Sesame, Coriander, and Pumpkin seed juice is truly remarkable. This company Activation Products, has managed to unlock the true potential energy from where all plant life begins and has made it bioavailable with true, unique, and highly sophisticated seed juice/oil extraction technology. This is one of the few ways where technology is actually offering a potential solution of getting missing elements in our diet in a safe way. It goes beyond the challenging, improperly handled, rancid inflammatory polyunsaturated fatty acids (PUFAs) mentioned before. We do need very small levels of these fatty acids, but packaged and extracted correctly in their suspended living state. We can get this from properly consuming and digesting enough nuts and seeds, but this tends to be somewhat inefficient and problematic for most. Experience true physical and emotional life enhancement in an edible way.

Pine Pollen

Traditionally used for more than 2,000 years, this substance has over 200 life-enhancing nutrients. It has a track record of strengthening, restoring, and building immunity. And with one of the highest concentrations of androgen (testosterone) building elements from any food, it also helps to balance hormonal profiles in the body.

Colostrum

Colostrum is the first milk secreted from the mammary glands of a mother mammal. True 6-hour colostrum is our original "first food." It has a complete profile of nutrients as it has naturally occurring growth factors, all essential amino acids, vitamins, minerals, fats, antioxidants, and rebuilding elements needed for robust health and a stronger immune system.

Bee Products

Bee pollen is an amino acid activator, one of nature's most complete foods, and a builder of structural components. Propolis is nature's penicillin and a natural antibiotic/protector without side effects. Royal Jelly is the queen's food and one of the most rejuvenating foods on the planet. Use wild honey with some of the highest levels of enzymes, B vitamins, and fructooligosaccharides to blend and round these 3 magical substances, and there's not much more to say on why to take them.

Blue Green Algae

Klamath Lake in Oregon is a very special place with lots of the planet's vital elements. Blue green algae harvested from such a place presents us with one of nature's richest sources of living chlorophyll. This assists with proper oxygenation of the body, natural self-cleansing abilities, neurotransmitter function, and potentiates an overall elevated state for the body spiritually and emotionally.

Medicinal Mushroom Blends

Immune modulating/protecting medicinal mushrooms have been used for thousands of years as decocted tea and powders to act as a shield and also a conductor of the intelligence of the planet. Some of the most profound ones are Chaga, Reishi, Cordyceps, Maiitake, and Shiitake.

One World Whey

Truly grass-fed, low temperature, non-acid-washed, whole whey protein. This is the most bioavailable concentrated protein source on the planet. It has one of the highest concentrations of glutathione – one of nature's most rebuilding and highest antioxidant type amino acids, which activates the interior of the cell and not just the outside. This particular protein has the ability to rebuild the body, enhance immunity, and assist in proper muscle-building and whole body recovery.

Should You Supplement?

So now that you have the proper whole food program down, possible biochemical typing via hair analysis and/or how you react to certain foods, you're drinking the best water, you're exercising properly, you've adapted many lifestyle changes, and you're taking some superfoods (or not;)), what the heck do you need supplements for? It's a good question that needs to be asked. We live in a far from ideal world where the soil is depleted, pollution abounds, we don't receive enough sunlight, and we have way too much stress. Every once in a while, supplementation may be needed to ASSIST – not to be solely relied upon. But not all supplements are created equal, and one has to have direction and go by specific biochemistry to choose correctly. This is why periodically performing the proper hair tissue analysis testing is helpful. This is what will let you know of any deficiencies, proper mineral ratios, metabolic indicators, and which specific supplements are needed and at what time. I also recommend caution from using any type of synthetic vitamin or mineral. It's always best to try whole food-based supplements first, that are pharmaceutical grade from living organisms. Be cautious about doctors' advice in this area.

Conclusion

There you have it – 10 years of self-experimentation, non-stop book learning, and in-the-field experience wrapped into a nice bundle that hopefully took 30 minutes or less to read. Remember, the intent behind this booklet is to plant seeds and hopefully offer a series of bullet-style points toward the attainment of robust health and vitality. There is a ton of health information out there, and I hope that this work provided an easy-to-follow skeleton so that your future lifestyle changes are meaningful and produce great results. Everyone has the ability, power, and access to achieving anything they want. Everybody today has the option of being truly healthy and living up to their full potential. I'm not perfect – far from it – and I'm still learning each day. Like everyone else, there are difficult, heavy days and there are some that are unbelievably amazing. It is my hope that we all strive to find balance, live with compassion, and move forward through our evolutionary path with respect and love for each other. Thank you for giving this book a chance, and I hope it brings to all of you a great deal of wisdom and avenues for further exploration.

Upgrade Your Life!

Thanks for reading my book! My goal is to provide a portal toward the attainment of robust and sovereign health. At Schotts Wellness, we are constantly staying up-to-date with the most cutting-edge lifestyle modification tools in order to improve our species. Visit our website at Schottswellness.com and join our quest, as we continue to bring forth practical rejuvenation strategies that will create evolutionary shifts, and a more balanced planet.

Share Your Feedback

Thank you again for reading this book. I do hope you found the information contained here to be helpful for your own personal health journey. I would really appreciate your feedback, so please take a moment to give a short review on Amazon. Your review will help me reach more readers, as well as help me in my future work and writing. Thank you again for reading and for taking the time to give your review!

Resources & Recipes

Rewilding: A Movement worth considering as the next phase after this book

I begin the resource page with Rewilding because it's a tool, but above all because it is a philosophical look toward where we are heading as a species. I believe it's of great importance to look at the bigger picture and break the chains of domestication. A blueprint toward becoming stronger and more feral beings is not only wise, but necessary. The following websites and links will open up a world toward a concept that is profound, and a new world of discovery we should all take part in.

- danielvitalis.com
- findaspring.com
- arthurhaines.com
- surthrival.com
- threelilyfarm.com
- gaiascouts.com

Living water systems

- Wherever applicable, www.findaspring.com
- Schottswellness.com; 786 505 6460 Miami, FL 33134

- www.pristinehydro.com
- Safe Drinking Bottles:
  http://www.lifefactory.com/catalog/adults;
  http://www.kleankanteen.com/

Emotional techniques, concepts, and websites

- http://www.birthintobeing.com/about_elena_tonetti_vladimirova
- Sacred Body Language: http://masterysystems.com
- Emotion Code: http://www.theemotioncode.com
- Body Talk: http://www.bodytalksystem.com
- Dr. John Demartini: https://drdemartini.com
- http://chriskehler.net/services.html

For Die-t trap & diet recovery:

- Schottswellness.com
- http://180degreehealth.com
- www.danielvitalis.com
- http://anthonycolpo.com

Proper testing & Bio chemical individualizations

- Hair tissue analysis: http://www.drgarrettsmith.com

For local farm fresh food & raw dairy:

- www.westonaprice.org look for your local chapter; if in South Florida, check out http://www.myhealthyfoodclub.com or BM Organics in Ft. Lauderdale tel:954.533.3282

- farmer's markets:
  - http://greenermiami.com/2011/01/top-10-farmers-markets-in-miami
  - https://www.glaserorganicfarms.com
  - http://makehealthyhappenmiami.com/html/farmers_markets.html
- Sustainability: polyfacefarms.com

Far & near Infrared Sauna

- Relax Sauna: http://oneradionetwork.com/uncategorized/sauna-landing-page
- Near infrared/ build it yourself:
  - http://www.drlwilson.com/SAUNAS/BUY%20OTHER%20SAUNAS.htm
  - http://drlwilson.com/SAUNAS/SAUNA%20PLANS.htm,
  - http://drlwilson.com/Books/saunabook.htm
- Clear Light infrared sauna: http://www.infraredsauna.com

Nutritional "fasting" with optimization ideas:

- Schottswellness.com; 786 505 6460 Miami, FL 33134

Lifestyle Management

Stress:

- Holo sync: https://www.centerpointe.com
- Profound Meditation-profoundmeditationprogram.com

Sleep:

- Book: *Lights Out* by TS Wiley
- Sleep monitoring systems: ZEO: http://amzn.to/1kCzLwW

FITBIT:

- http://amzn.to/1kCzRof

Bulbs & glasses:

- https://www.lowbluelights.com/index.asp; google- Uvex S1933X Skyper Safety Eyeware

Sleep CD:

- Delta Sleep System: http://amzn.to/1yxUweg

To install in your computer:

- Flux: http://stereopsis.com/flux

Assists in going to sleep faster:

- GoLite: http://amzn.to/VlbgZw
- Nightwave- http://www.nightwave.com

Other things to consider:

- Air-o-swiss: http://amzn.to/1rtgZGQ

Poppy extract:

- http://amzn.to/VlbqQx

Melatonin (temporary solution):

- http://www.iherb.com/Source-Naturals-Melatonin-3-mg-240-Tablets/1314

Exercise

- Anything that will get the body moving and resisting.

- Yoga, rebounding, walking, sprints, high-intensity interval training, martial arts, weight or body-weight training, sports.

Sites:

- Natural Movement: movnat.com; idoportal.com; google Scott Sonnen

- *True martial arts (mostly for locals in South Florida): Steve Zalut sangwa3@gmail.com*

- Also Krav Maga is cool as heck

- Isometrics: http://www.isometric-training.com

- Slow burn/ Akum's

- Stretching:
  - Bob Cooley: https://www.thegeniusofflexibility.com
  - Ki Hara: http://ki-hara.com

- Proper lifting & Miami gyms: crossfitsoulmiami.com http://www.primalfitmiami.com

- Rebounders: http://oneradionetwork.com/health-articles/reboundair

- Five Finger Shoes: http://www.vibramfivefingers.com/index.htm

EMF (electro magnetic frequencies) and Health:

- http://jackkruse.com

- http://www.michaelneuert.com

- One of the best ways to protect the body from frequencies from cell phones and computers is to get the devices as far away from the body as possible, especially the brain. So one of the best strategies for cell phone use is to purchase an ear piece with microphone that ideally has a hollow tube (not a blue tooth wireless ear piece – this is worse, since it emits EMFs like a mini antennae in your ear). You can find this at mercola.com. If the air tube breaks, as these sometimes do, get the ear piece designed for your phone and add an extra diffuser box to the cable found at blockemf.com or lessemf.com.

- The other investment for EMF protection is to get a tri field meter which measures electric, magnetic, and micro wave emissions in your home, so that you can move your bed or other furnishings accordingly (do this only if you will actually use it consistently and have the extra cash).

Sites:

- http://www.electricsense.com/988/where-is-the-place-you-absolutely-must-start-if-you-want-to-protect-yourself-from-electromagnetic-radiation

- blockemf.com

- http://www.radmeters.com/Cornet-ED25G-ssm.html

- http://www.stetzerelectric.com/

- http://antennasearch.com/default.asp

- http://microwavenews.com/

- http://refusesmartmeters.com/

- http://smartmeterguard.com

Environment/ Healthy Home:

- Book: *Super Natural Home* by Beth Greer
  - amzn.to/1AhcHrs
  - http://supernaturalmom.com
- http://hbelc.org/, http://www.monolithic.com
- Safe Drinking Bottles
  - http://www.lifefactory.com/catalog/adults
  - http://www.kleankanteen.com
- Non-toxic cookware:
  - http://earthshiftproducts.com/Products.aspx?comcode=AC&plinid=CERAM&plnmain=KITCHENWARE

- o http://www.saladmaster.com/display/router.aspx
- Clean Air:
  - o http://www.mosonatural.com/
  - o http://www.marycordaro.com/products/air_cleaners.html
- Smart Meters:
  - o http://refusesmartmeters.com/page24.html
  - o http://www.radmeters.com/Cornet-ED25G-ssm.html
- Shower Filter:
  - o http://www.santeforhealth.com/shopexd.asp?id=439
  - o http://www.aquasana.com/category.php?category_id=2, http://www.rainshowermfg.com
- Non Toxic Paint: http://www.ecospaints.net
- Natural house cleaners:
  - o http://www.drbronner.com
  - o book: amzn.to/1rthvES
- LED Bulbs:
  - o amzn.to/1uxDsri
  - o http://goo.gl/WcmVRc
- Plants: http://greenplantsforgreenbuildings.org
- Clothing: http://www.vivaterra.com
- Non-toxic toys: http://achildsdream.com

Superfoods & staples

- Marine Phytoplankton: http://www.activationproducts.com/store/oceans-alive-30ml?AFFID=113981

- Panaseeda seed oil: http://www.activationproducts.com?AFFID=113981

- Colostrum, Pine Pollen, Medicinal Mushrooms: http://www.1shoppingcart.com/app/?af=1521095

- Honey Products: local or health food stores

- Blue Green Algae: e3live.com

- Other Medicinal Mushroom Products:
  - jingherbs.com
  - dragonherbs.com

- Protein: One World Whey

Books: Whole food perspectives and Traditional food preparation

- *Nourishing Traditions* by Sally Fallon

- *Catching Fire: How Cooking Made Us Human* by Richard Wrangham

- *The Vegetarian Myth* by Leirre Keith

- *The Paleo Solution* by Robb Wolf

- *The Primal Blueprint* by Mark Sisson

Great food blogs

- threelilyfarm.com
- http://thebarefootcook.com
- http://www.anorganicwife.com
- http://paleoista.com
- http://thehealthyfoodie.com

Nutrition (real food oriented) certification schools:

- Nutritional Therapy Association nutritionaltherapy.com
- Institute for Integrative Nutrition integrativenutrition.com
- pricepottenger.com

Probiotics:

- Sauerkraut (homemade, farmer's market, health food stores)
- Kimchee
- Yogurt, kefir
- Coconut water kefir; kefir starter:
- www.bodyecologydiet.com

Herbs:

- mountainroseherbs.com

Food & Health Politics:

- naturalnews.com

Movies:

- Zeitgeist
- Hungry for Change: http://www.hungryforchange.tv
- Farmageddon: http://farmageddonmovie.com
- Food Inc.: http://www.takepart.com/foodinc

Great websites:

- danielvitalis.com
- oneradionetwork.com
- 180degreeshealth.com
- naturalnews.com
- westonaprice.org
- anthonycolpo.com
- thepaleosolution.com
- marksdailyapple.com
- mercola.com

Appendix A: Breakfast

(Check for recipes & more ideas on schottwellness.com)

- Fruit crumble
- Veggie omelet
- Smoothies and shakes
- Gluten Free waffles
- Gluten Free pancakes

Appendix B: Lunch

(Check for recipes & more ideas on schottwellness.com)

- Wild salmon with cauliflower rice and brussels sprouts
- Bison burger with sweet potato fries
- Ground chicken burger with easy onion rings
- Portobello cheese olive oil sandwich with sweet potato, or cauliflower mash
- Grass-fed burger with yuca fries and suero
- Curry chicken breast
- Fish stew
- Chicken stew

Appendix C: Dinners

(Check for recipes & more ideas on schottwellness.com)
All lunch meals work here and the following are lighter meals:

- Cottage cheese and rotated veggies
- Small portion wild rice with olive oil and veggies
- Mushroom/ baby bok choy Stir fry
- Steamed veggies with olive oil and 1 slice of toast
- Veggie soup (onion, cauliflower, crucifers)
- Purée soups (butternut, spinach, asparagus)
- Caprese salad
- Bruschetta salad
- Homemade veggie pizza

Recipes:

Cauliflower rice

- 1 head cauliflower
- 2-4 tbs. grass-fed butter, ghee or olive oil
- 1- 2 tbs. nutritional yeast (optional)
- 1 tsp. sea salt
- 2 tsp. onion powder (optional)
- Curly parsley finely chopped

Lightly steam cauliflower

Place cauliflower, butter, nutritional yeast, in food processor and lightly chop on and off a few time to get consistency of rice

Place in a bowl, add other ingredients and mix with a spatula

---

Cauliflower mash

- 1 head cauliflower
- 2-4 tbs. grass fed butter, ghee or olive oil
- 1- 2 tbs. nutritional yeast (optional)
- 1 tsp. sea salt
- 2 tsp. onion powder
- 1/2 tsp. garlic powder or 1 small clove

Lightly steam cauliflower

Place cauliflower and remaining ingredients in food processor; chop until you reach a mashed potato consistency

Note: for **Sweet Potato Mash** and **Butternut Squash Mash,** do the same but cook the sweet potato until soft. And you can peel both of these before steaming.

Beef kebabs

- 1 4oz- 6oz grass-fed sirloin steak
- 1/2 bell pepper
- 1/2 red onion
- 4 cherry tomatoes
- 1 yellow squash

Cut sirloin into cubes, slice vegetable into squares except for cherry tomato; take bamboo skewer and place one piece of onion, one piece of bell pepper, one piece of squash and one piece of the sirloin onto the skewer tightly – repeat as many times as the length of the skewer allows and finish with a cherry tomato on top

Place on a pan or grill and add butter, Ghee, or olive oil with a brush and season accordingly with salt, cumin as you cook

Bison butternut chili

- 1/4 to 1 lb. ground bison, depending on quantity desired

- 1/2 butternut squash, cubed into small pieces – skin can be peeled if desired

- 1/4 onion

- 1 tomato

- organic tomato sauce or paste

- 2-4 tbs. butter or ghee

- 1 handful cilantro

- 1-2 tsp. chili powder

- 1-2 tap. paprika

- 1-2 tsp. salt

In a pot, lightly steam butternut squash cubes. You can cook some sprouted lentils or a bit of black beans with this, if desired, but not necessary.

In a separate pan, sauté onion in butter, ghee or Olive oil, add chopped tomatoes, add bison and cook until bison is almost done. Add this mix into the pot with the butternut. Add spices, salt and tomato sauce or paste. For sauce, use anywhere from 1/4 to 3/4 of a cup, depending on quantity. Cook on low until desired consistency.

Grass-fed stuffed peppers

- 1/4 to 1 lb. ground beef, depending on quantity desired
- 1-4 red bell peppers
- 1/4 onion
- 1 tomato
- organic tomato sauce or paste
- 2-4 tbs. butter or ghee
- 1-2 tsp. paprika
- 1-2 tsp. salt
- 1-2 cups pre-made cauliflower rice

Sauté onion in butter, ghee or Olive oil, add chopped tomatoes, add beef and cook until beef is almost done. In a bowl, add beef with the tomato sauce and cauliflower rice and spices.

Slice peppers on top, core and place beef cauliflower mix into the peppers. Cook in oven at 350 for about 1- 1.5 hours.

If you desire an easier way, simply mix all ingredients in a bowl, stuff the peppers and put it in a slow cooker on low for about 4 to 6 hours

Note: these can be made with ground turkey, lamb, or bison, as well

Slow cooked Peach BBQ spare ribs

- 1- 3 lbs. of beef short ribs, boneless or bone-in
- 1/4 to 1/2 red onion, sliced
- 2 stalks celery, diced
- 1-2 carrots, diced
- 1/2 cup water
- 2 tbs. apple cider vinegar
- 1 tsp. paprika

Peach glaze

- 1-2 peaches cored
- 1-2 tbs. Honey
- Pinch of salt
- 1/2 tsp. Mesquite
- 1 tsp. Coconut aminos
- 1 tbs. Olive oil

Place all ingredients for peach glaze in a blender or food processor and blend.

Line the bottom of slow cooker with 1/2 of the veggies. Brush ribs on both sides generously with peach glaze and save the rest for when ribs are finished. Place short ribs on top of veggies.

Mix remaining veggies over ribs and cover crock pot. Cook on low for 8 hours.

Pumpkin beef burgers

- 1/4 pumpkin, steamed and puréed, or 1 can organic pumpkin

- 1/2 lbs. grass-fed ground beef

- 1 tsp. paprika

- 1 tsp. palm sugar (optional)

- Pinch of mesquite

- Salt to taste

Mix puréed pumpkin with beef and all ingredients. Add an egg yolk, if desired, for better burger consistency. Make into patties and "grill" in a pan pre-oiled with butter, ghee, or red palm oil.

Wrap with lightly steamed de-stemmed collard greens, sauerkraut or kimchee and sprouts

---

Grass fed roast with veggies

- 1-2 lbs. chuck roast or meat of choice

- 2-3 carrots, peeled (optional) and sliced

- 1 large red onion, sliced

- 1 head of broccoli, cut into florets

- 1/2 purple cabbage, sliced

- 2-3 cloves of garlic, halved

- 1/2 to 1 cup beef broth, if available

- Salt to taste

Place onion, garlic and 1/2 carrots on bottom of crock pot with beef broth or same amount of water. Roast on low, covered, overnight or 6 hours. Place all remaining vegetables on and around the roast 1-2 hours before roast is done. Cover and cook until finished

Note: this can be done with lamb roast and you can add cumin and 1/8 gram masala for a different and delicious flavor.

Grass-fed steak burritos with Mexican-style salad

- 4-6 oz. grass fed steak
- 1/4 red bell pepper
- 1/4 cup red chopped onion
- Handful of cilantro
- 1-2 tbs. Coconut liquid aminos
- Chili pepper, paprika and salt to taste

Sauté veggies in ghee or red palm oil until golden. Add thinly sliced steak and cooked to desired consistency. Right before finishing the steak, add cilantro and coconut aminos and condiments.

Wrap in de-stemmed collard, lightly steamed cabbage, large romaine leaf or natural tortilla of choice.

Salad is simply greens, sprouts, homemade guacamole, with same spices, olive oil and apple cider vinegar; handful of purple corn chips, if tolerated and desired, can be crushed into the salad, as well.

Zucchini pasta with grass-fed meatballs

- 2 zucchini or yellow squash

- 1/2- 1 lbs. ground grass-fed beef

- 1-2 cloves garlic

- 1/4 C chopped onion

- 1/2 C tomato sauce

- 1-2 tsp. wild raw honey

- Olive oil

- Salt to taste

Cut ends of zucchini and make into spaghetti noodles using spirooli or noodle slicer of choice. Cover the zucchini spaghetti with lots of sea salt, place on top of strainer over a bowl and let water drain overnight. Next day, rinse the salt off with water.

In a pan, sauté onion in butter, ghee or olive oil, add chopped onion and garlic and cook until golden. Add preformed meatballs and cook until beef is halfway done. Add tomato sauce and remaining ingredients, turning meatballs and cook on low until desired consistency. Add the zucchini pasta while cooking or sauté in a separate pan with butter, and serve on a dish with meatballs & sauce on top.

Lamb vegetable loaf

- 1/2- 1 lbs. ground lamb
- 1 serving kale and/or collards
- 2-3 eggs
- 1 zucchini
- Salt to taste
- 1/4 tsp each cumin, dried parsley, and curry

Chop kale and/or collards and zucchini in a food processor or finely chopped with a knife.

In a bowl, crack eggs, beat with a whisk and add lamb, chopped veggies and condiments. Mix by hand and place in a loaf pan. Cook in a pre-heated oven at 375 for 1- 1.5 hours, or until fork goes in and out of loaf smoothly with no residue.

Accompany with salad and/or sweet potato mash

Turkey meatballs with sweet potato linguini

- 1 sweet potato
- 1/2- 1 lbs. ground turkey
- 1-2 cloves garlic
- 1/4 C chopped onion
- 2-4 tbs. Olive oiler butter
- Salt to taste

Peel sweet potato and slice thinly with a mandolin into lasagna-type sheets. With a chef's knife, slice into linguini. Cook in a pan with butter, ghee or olive oil until soft.

In a pan, sauté onion in butter, ghee or olive oil, add chopped onion and garlic and cook until golden. Add preformed meatballs and cook until turkey halfway done. Add remaining ingredients and cook on low until desired consistency.

Add the cooked sweet potato linguini while cooking or sauté in a separate pan with butter and serve on a dish with meatballs and butter on top.

Slow-cooked chicken with cauliflower & pea "rice"

- 1 whole chicken or leg and thigh
- sprigs fresh rosemary
- 1 lemon, zested, halved and juiced
- ¼ cup organic honey
- 1 tbsp. Dijon mustard
- ½ white onion, quartered
- 3 cloves of garlic, peeled
- Salt and pepper to taste

Season the outside and inside of the chicken generously with salt and pepper. Set the chicken in the crock pot.

Chop up 2 sprigs of rosemary. Place the chopped rosemary, lemon zest, lemon juice, honey, and Dijon mustard in a pan on low to soften honey and mix seasonings well. Place the remaining sprig of rosemary, quartered onions, garlic, and lemon halves inside the cavity of the chicken. Brush the honey Dijon mixture all over the chicken, coating heavily. Cook on low in the crock pot for 6-8 hours.

When removing the chicken from the crock pot, it will want to fall apart. Either remove carefully to keep intact, or let the meat fall off the bone.

Make cauliflower rice and add to sautéed peas in butter.

Ground turkey sandwich with purple potato fries

- 1/4-1 lbs. ground turkey
- 1/2 tsp. cumin
- 1/2- 1 tsp. oregano
- Salt to taste
- 1 egg yolk
- 1 purple onion
- 1-3 purple potatoes

Slice onion thinly and add to buttered pan until golden and caramelized.

Mix ground turkey, egg yolk and spices in a bowl, form into patties and cook in a pre-oiled pan on medium heat. Flip until desired cooking terms.

Wrap in de-stemmed collard wrap with sliced tomato and caramelized onion. Add mustard and non-soy mayo.

Slice purple potato and make into fries with coconut oil or baked in oven.

Farm chicken breast collards and avocado salsa

- 1 chicken breast
- 2-4 tbs. butter
- 1 avocado
- 1/4. C onions chopped
- 4 cherry tomatoes chopped finely
- 1 tbs. olive oil
- 1 tsp. apple cider vinegar
- Salt to taste

Butter pan while steaming de-stemmed collard greens. Place chicken breast in butter and add salt and other desired condiments as desired until chicken breast is cooked fully. Once collards are well-steamed, place in a food processor with butter and 1/2 tsp. sea salt. Pulse until pate consistency.

Cut avocado into cubes and mix in a bowl with vinegar, oil, salt to taste and onion and tomato. Top the chicken breast with avocado salsa and enjoy with collards.

Chicken Kebabs with cauliflower tabuleh no-bean hummus

- 1 4oz- 6oz chicken breast
- 1/2 bell pepper
- 1/2 red onion
- 4 cherry tomatoes

- 1 yellow squash

Cut chicken into cubes, slice vegetables into squares except for cherry tomato; take bamboo skewer and place one piece of onion, one piece of bell pepper, one piece of squash and one piece of chicken onto the skewer tightly - repeat as many times as the length of the skewer and finish with a cherry tomato on top

Place on a pan or grill and add butter, Ghee, or olive oil with a brush and season accordingly with salt, cumin as you cook

---

Cauliflower Tabuleh

- 1 head cauliflower
- 2-4 tbs. olive oil
- 1/2 C chopped tomato
- 1/2 C chopped onion
- 1-2 lemons juiced
- 1 tsp. sea salt
- 1 bunch curly parsley, finely-chopped

Lightly steam cauliflower

Place cauliflower in food processor and lightly chop on and off a few time to get consistency of rice

Place cauliflower in a bowl, add other ingredients and mix with a spatula

Brazil Nut Hummus (makes 1.5 cups):

- ½ C Brazil nuts
- ½ C Pine nuts
- 3 heaping tbs. raw tahini
- 4 ½ tbs. lemon juice
- 2 tbs. olive oil
- 1 tsp. sun-dried sea salt
- ½ clove of garlic
- ½ C charged water

Place nuts in a Cuisinart food processor with an S blade and grind them into a thick paste. Add the remaining ingredients and pulse a few more times.

Note: Always use a rubber spatula to scrape the sides of the processor and get an even mixture.

Hearty Vegetable chicken Soup

- 1/2 C chopped onion
- 1/4 C chopped bell pepper
- 3 carrots
- 2-4 tbs. grass-fed butter or ghee
- 1-3 purple potato
- Yucca (optional)
- 1/2 purple cabbage

- 2-4. C broth
- 1 chicken leg and thigh
- 1 tsp. salt
- 1 tsp. paprika
- 1/2 tsp. cumin
- 1/4 tsp. turmeric

Sauté onions, bell peppers in butter or ghee in a soup pot until caramelized, add chicken stock and chicken and cook for about 1-2 hours on medium/ low until chicken softens; add the vegetables and remaining ingredients and cook on medium until veggies are cooked and very slightly crispy.

Stuffed Portobello Caps with turkey and sweet potato fries

- 1-2 Portobello caps
- 1/4-1 lbs. ground turkey
- 1/4 C chopped onion
- 1/2 tsp. chili powder
- Salt to taste
- 1 sweet potato
- Coconut oil

Take Portobello caps and with a spoon, scrape inside until hollow. Place the mushroom aside and in a separate pan sauté onions until golden. Add turkey until almost fully cooked. Add scraped Portobello and spices until everything is well cooked. Set to the side in a bowl and "grill" Portobello caps in same skillet until slightly soft. Add turkey mix on top.

Peel and slice sweet potato and make into fries with coconut oil or baked in oven.

Chicken chop with cauliflower curry rice and butternut cubes

- 1 chicken breast
- Butter and salt to taste

Place chicken breast in butter and add salt and other desired condiments as desired until chicken breast is cooked fully. Chop into cubes, and set aside to go over cauliflower curry rice.

Cauliflower curry rice

- 1 head cauliflower
- 2-4 tbs. coconut oil
- 1 tsp. sea salt
- 1 tsp. curry powder
- 2 tsp. onion powder (optional)

Lightly steam cauliflower

Place cauliflower in food processor and lightly chop on and off a few times to get consistency of rice.

Place in a bowl, add other ingredients and mix with a spatula.

Butternut Cubes

- 1/2 butternut squash peeled and cubed
- 2-4 tbs. coconut oil

Lightly steam butternut until almost fully soft. In a separate pan, heat coconut oil on medium, add the butternut, salt to taste and add pinch of cinnamon.

Herbed baked chicken over spaghetti squash

- 1 whole chicken or 1/2 chicken
- 2 tbsp. grass-fed butter, melted
- 1 tbsp. sage
- 1 sprig thyme
- 1 sprig rosemary
- 1/2 lemon
- Salt to taste

Preheat oven to 400° F. Lightly rinse chicken and squeeze and rub with the 1/2 lemon. Coat bottom of pan with butter and melt with most of the chopped herbs and salt. Rub and pour all over chicken pieces and remaining seasoning.

Bake for 30 minutes; reduce heat to 350° F. Continue baking for 15-30 minutes or until chicken reaches an internal temperature of at least 165° F.

To crisp the skin, broil chicken for the last 5 minutes.

Spaghetti Squash

- 1 spaghetti squash, halved lengthwise and seeded
- 2 tablespoons butter or ghee

Preheat oven to 350 degrees F (175 degrees C). Lightly grease a baking sheet.

Place spaghetti squash with cut sides down on the prepared baking sheet, and bake 30 minutes in the preheated oven, or until a sharp knife can be inserted with only a little resistance. Remove squash from oven and set aside to cool enough to be easily handled.

Use a large spoon or fork to scoop the stringy pulp from the squash and place in a medium bowl. Toss with butter and desired spices.

Chicken cacciatore over "pasta"

- 1 lb. chicken thighs
- ¼ cup coconut oil, melted
- 1 cup red onion, diced
- 1 red bell pepper, roasted and diced
- 1/4 Serrano pepper, roasted and diced
- 1 tsp. ground cumin
- 1 tsp. paprika

- 1/4 tsp. allspice

- 1/4 tsp. nutmeg

- 2 medium chopped tomatoes with juice

- 1/2 cup water (or broth of choice)

- 2 tbsp. red wine

- 4 ounces organic tomato paste

- 1 cup organic pumpkin puree

Heat coconut oil in a large Dutch oven over medium-high heat. Add chicken and brown on all sides, about 6-8 minutes. Remove to platter. Add red onions to the oil in the Dutch oven and sauté until tender, approximately 5 minutes. Add peppers, cinnamon stick, cumin, paprika, allspice, nutmeg, and cloves. Stir constantly for 2 minutes. Add in tomatoes and water, and mix well. Place all of the chicken in this sauce, cover, and simmer over medium-low heat until chicken is very tender, approximately 30-40 minutes.

Transfer chicken to a platter and tent with aluminum foil to keep warm. Add red wine vinegar, tomato paste, and pumpkin puree to the sauce. Simmer and stir until reduced to sauce consistency, about 10 minutes. Season with salt and pepper to taste. Serve over a bed of spaghetti squash or sweet potato pasta.

Honey Mustard Baked Chicken Thighs

- 1 chicken leg and thigh combo
- 2 tbsp. grass-fed butter, melted
- 1/4 C clean honey mustard or mustard with 2 tbs. wild honey
- 1 lemon
- Salt to taste

Preheat oven to 400° F. Lightly rinse chicken and squeeze and rub with the lemon. Coat bottom of pan with butter and melt honey mustard. Rub and pour all over chicken pieces. Note: ideally, leave marinating overnight.

Bake for 30 minutes; reduce the heat to 350° F. Continue baking for 15-30 minutes or until chicken reaches an internal temperature of at least 165° F.

Turkey Bacon apple-stuffed chicken breasts

- 1-2 boneless, skinless chicken breasts
- 4 slices nitrate-free turkey bacon
- 1 apple
- 1-2 tbs. butter
- Salt and pepper to taste

Sauté apple and butter with a pinch of salt until soft.

Preheat oven to 375° F. Carefully butterfly open chicken breasts, ensuring not to slice all the way through.

Season the inside of the breasts with salt and pepper. Spread buttered apple to taste inside of the filleted breasts. Fold the chicken breasts closed back onto themselves and wrap two slices of bacon around each. Secure the bacon to itself and the chicken with a toothpick.

Place the chicken in a Pyrex baking dish and bake for 30 minutes or until chicken is almost done.

Remove chicken, set oven to broil on high and then place chicken on the top shelf of the oven for 5-10 minutes to get the bacon nice and brown. Serve with your veggies of choice and enjoy.

For **turkey bacon wrapped tahini/ sun dried tomato breast,** do the same but use tahini and sun-dried tomato to taste as stuffing.

Lemon Dijon Chicken with cauliflower mango couscous

- 1 chicken breast
- 1/4 C Dijon mustard
- 1 lemon, juiced
- 1 tbs. olive oil
- 1 tsp. lemon zest
- Salt to taste

Mix all condiments, lemon juice and zest, salt and mustard, in a bowl and add mixture to chicken breast; marinate overnight. Grill to desired consistency, using all marinade.

Cauliflower mango couscous

- 1 head cauliflower
- 2-4 tbs. olive oil
- 1 mango finely chopped
- 1 tsp. sea salt
- 1/2 lemon juiced

Lightly steam cauliflower

Place cauliflower in food processor and lightly chop on and off a few time to get consistency of couscous

Place in a bowl, add other ingredients and mix with a spatula

---

BBQ slow-cooked chicken

- 1 whole chicken
- 1 white onion, sliced
- 2 tsp. paprika
- 1 tsp. sea salt
- 1 tsp. onion powder
- 1 tsp. Mesquite
- 1 tsp. dried thyme
- 1 tsp. white pepper
- 1 tsp. cayenne
- ½ tsp. garlic powder

Line the bottom of the crock pot with the sliced onions. Place the chicken in the crock pot on top of the onions.

Combine all remaining ingredients in a bowl and mix well. Rub the mixture over the entire chicken - in and out and thick.

Place the lid on crock pot and cook on low for 6 hours or until chicken is done.

Sweet Potato Hash

- 1 sweet potato
- 2-4 tbs. coconut oil
- 1 tbs. potato starch (optional)

Peel sweet potato and shred with mandolin into thin strips. Mix with starch into patties and cook with oil.

Vietnamese Spring Roll

- 4-6 rice or tapioca paper rolls
- Bok choy, celery, nappa cabbage, shredded carrots
- 2 tbs. olive oil
- 1 tsp. apple cider vinegar or plumb vinegar
- Ground meat of choice (optional)
- 1/4 tsp. ginger
- Coconut aminos to taste

- Salt to taste

Make stir fry with all ingredients except rice or tapioca wraps. Take the wraps and place in a large dish with water to soften. Pat dry, pour small amounts of stir fry and wrap according to directions on the pack.

Tortilla Recipe:
Makes 15
- 1.5 C coconut or nut milk
- 1.5 C apple
- 1 tsp. sea salt
- 3 tbs. coconut oil
- 2.5 C water
- 2 C ground flax or chia

Blend all ingredients except flax or chia. Pour liquid in a bowl, add flax or chia and whisk. Place about 1 ladle-sized tortilla on teflex sheet and shape into tortilla. Dehydrate for 8 hours, flip and dehydrate for 3-4 hours.

About the Author

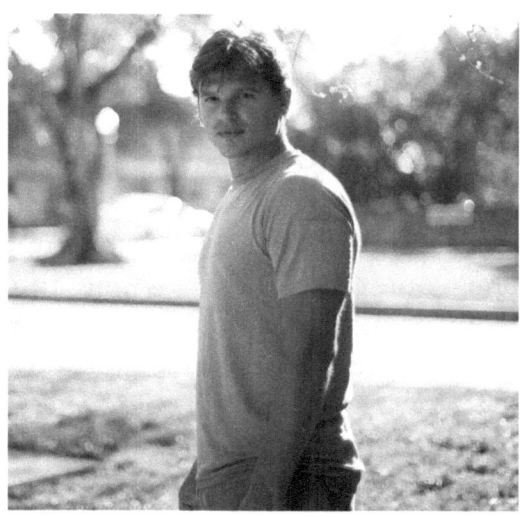

My whole life – as a boy growing up in my hometown, and now as an adult – I have always intuitively known that my mission has been to spread love and assist humanity in overcoming limits and breaking new ground. Seeing the inequities of the class system alive and well in third-world Colombia, a passion to help humanity bubbled up inside from a very young age. As an entrepreneur in the health field, I have learned the value of hard work and excellence in everything I put forth. I pride myself on my high level of ethics and integrity in this over-saturated and confusing field of health and nutrition.

Throughout my evolution in the health field, I have run the gamut of all diets and nutritional disciplines – both time-tested and newly developed. This has brought me to a unique and more holistic place from where to educate the public on all matters of nutrition. As a gifted whole food chef, my skill exemplifies the standard of optimal health, as well as gourmet cuisine. I am continually engaged in self-study and I am constantly absorbing new information. After 10 years of serving in the health field, and five years of being a health-food restaurant owner and general manager in Miami, Fla., I understand that this is still a very young and somewhat uncharted field. My wisdom increases with each passing day, and I appreciate all there is to learn, as I realize there is always some new facet to immerse myself in, and there are always ways to improve.

I have exposed myself to the wide spectrum of diets and food disciplines out there. I have gone through all the extremes – from being "nourished" by the SAD (Standard American Diet), veganism, vegetarianism, raw vegan, low-carb paleo diet, low fat diet, RBTI, blood type diet, primal diet and paleo. I do not have the next diet fad du jour with my name splattered all over complementary supplements to offer you. Why? Because after all these years, arduous research, and experimentations, I have found balance in eating real food in a sensible and very consciously, omnivorous manner. I believe we all benefit most from listening to our own bodies and understanding that biology is the greatest gauge. I also take advantage of some sound modern diagnostic technologies to monitor bio markers, and all biological levels, so as to minimize the guessing games. I am always on the cutting edge of whole body and nutritional programs. Be on the cutting edge along with me and visit www.schottswellness.com. Own your health!

www.ingramcontent.com/pod-product-compliance
Lightning Source LLC
Chambersburg PA
CBHW050507290526
45786CB00006B/2468